Praise

"Dr. Gail Jackson has guided me with grace from fibroids to fabulousness! Absolutely Fabulous is an example of her wealth of experience and plethora of knowledge in hormonal balance, and through the many chapters of womanhood, she has been a game changer in my health, wellness, and happiness! She is more than a doctor. She is a confidant, counselor, advocate, and friend. I am forever grateful for her gift in inspiring and guiding me to live a well-balanced and 'Absolutely Fabulous' LIFE!" **Wendy Raquel Robinson**, Two-Time Emmy Award Winning Producer and NAACP Actress and Director

"Imagine finding a doctor who not only possesses exceptional medical expertise but also exudes genuine care and compassion towards her patients. That's exactly what I experienced with Dr. Jackson. From delivering my son 18 years ago to continuously seeking out innovative treatments, she truly goes above and beyond to ensure her patients look and feel their best. She's a true lifesaver. Absolutely Fabulous is a must-read." **Kandy Isley,** Singer, Songwriter, Record Executive, Manager, and CEO of Ronald Isley Liquid Gold Spirits

"One of the best turning points in my life was when I crossed paths with Dr. Gail Jackson. I love knowing I have someone who truly understands how to make the aging process better! My hormone health has given me my youth back. Not to boast too much, but my sweetheart says the quality of my life has changed, and for that, I'm forever grateful!!!! Absolutely Fabulous can do the same for you!" **Angela Gibbs**, Actress, Acting Coach, and Director

"Every woman needs a Dr. Gail. She is like a General leading you to victory over hormonal health after 40, and Absolutely Fabulous is a look into her magic. Before her treatment, I had no energy, gained

weight, experienced brain fog, and struggled to sleep at night. My days were exhausting, and my nights were restless. Thanks to Dr. Gail's treatment, I now feel energized, well-rested, and revitalized." **Tasha Smith**, Director and Actress

"Dr Gail changed my life. I didn't know what was wrong with me. I just didn't feel like myself. Once I got the hormone replacement, I felt like I could think clearer, and I was able to lose weight. I was sleeping better. I wasn't cranky. I felt like myself again. I'm grateful for her. Absolutely Fabulous is a must-read for women 40 and older." **Erica Campbell**, Grammy Award-Winning Gospel Artist

"Absolutely Fabulous should be on every woman's bookshelf, regardless of her age. Reading Dr. Gail Jackson's insights and advice is like having a conversation with a friend who sees your whole self, brings out the best in you, and allows you to really shine. As women, we dedicate so much of our lives to the care of others, to our careers, or to simply getting through the day. Absolutely Fabulous is a definitive guide on learning to embrace the transcendent and life-affirming impact of self-care. Packed with tips, strategies, and knowledge Dr. Jackson has gleaned over decades of providing expert medical care to thousands of women. This book will reinvigorate, motivate, and inspire you to embrace your most fabulous self." **Areva Martin,** Esq., USA Today and Wall Street Journal Bestselling Author

"I feel so grateful to have had access to such a wonderful clinician, Dr Gail Jackson. I began as her patient in my early 20s, and thanks to her evolved practice, in my early 50s, I continue to have the fortune of being her patient and friend. I've always felt cared for and in good hands. As I continue to live life, I know that I have someone to confide in to guide me in living the vital life that I will always want to live! Thanks Dr J!" **Queen Latifah** Grammy Award-Winning Rapper, Singer, and Actress

ABSOLUTELY FABULOUS

GAIL N. JACKSON MD

DEDICATION

To my mom, Velma Jackson, who suffered silently and courageously through abrupt surgical menopause without any offer of support.

To my daughter, Jennifer Smart-Abbey MD, and her generation who will be armed with all of the information and options available to them.

TABLE OF CONTENTS

INTRODUCTION

We stand on the shoulders of the generation of women before us. They did so much with so little care and attention for and to them. Self-care was never considered, let alone any talk about balancing hormones. In the majority of our parents' and grandparents' relationships, a woman's role was solely one of homemaking and caregiving. She beamed with pride relishing the lives she was able to mold. There were very few opportunities or interests outside of the home, and those available offered very little pay. The highest profession a woman could achieve was probably in the field of education. However, times have changed, and women today pride themselves in the lives they shape and mold and the businesses they run. Age fifty is not what it used to be. It now heralds a new life with new opportunities and responsibilities. With this new life, women no longer accept the limitation of the symptoms of perimenopause and menopause and its sequelae as their fate.

Over 15 years ago, many of my patients were miserable. They felt hot, fragile, irritated, and cranky as soon as their body started to go through "the change." In her book, *I Am Too Young for This*, Suzanne Somers affectionately depicts the miseries of menopause through "The Seven Dwarfs of Menopause." From its creator, Alison Bourne, these menacing little creatures are dubbed: ITCHY, BITCHY, BLOATY, FORGETFUL, SWEATY, SLEEPY, and PSYCHO. Sound familiar? I cannot fathom a more suitable depiction or stress enough that you are not alone or crazy for feeling any of these symptoms. A sizable amount of my patients complained about experiencing these symptoms, and I noticed they were starting younger. What used to be common in women fifty and over is now starting in women who are in their early to mid-forties.

Like my patients, when the symptoms of perimenopause and menopause became almost unbearable, your first thought was probably to bring this up to your OBGYN. We are trained to help women at many different stages, so we must know how to help you feel better and more like yourself again. As a doctor, the solutions available and offered by traditional Western medicine quickly disappointed me because they simply didn't work and were not safe. My patients were not getting relief, and you probably are not either. So, I turned to integrative functional medicine and found the solutions I sought there. I then made it my life's ambition to deepen and widen my scope of knowledge. I wanted to help my precious suffering patients and, selfishly, to have all the solutions when the time came that I would need them for myself. With every resource at my disposal, I eventually found my way into bio-identical hormone balancing.

Many practitioners offer hormone therapies. So, what makes me different? For starters, not only am I a diplomate of the American Board of Obstetrics and Gynecology (meaning I am board certified in obstetrics and gynecology), I am also a thirty-year member of the obstetrical and gynecological medical staff at the prestigious Cedars-Sinai Medical Center. I have the most extensive and exclusive Western traditional medical information and resources available to me, and I have garnered all of the Western medicine credentials available in my specialty. To be frank, I am an expert in my field, and my life and the lives of my patients show the successful results of the work I get to do.

What I am sharing with you in this book is not in the required readings for medical students, nor is it found in the traditional and revered texts and journals that serve as the foundation of our gynecological specialty. Bio-identical hormone balancing enables a woman to maintain her exuberance and productivity as she transitions through perimenopause and menopause. Honestly, I can admit that I was a nay-sayer, along with the many other gynecologists who dismissed bio-identical hormones as unfounded and not supported by medical science. Before I started my research, there was a doctor in the area already looking into bio-identical hormones, and I thought he was a quack. Clearly, whatever he was doing could not be right. I know, I know—I was fine being one of those traditional practitioners until I could not take the misery of my patients anymore and I felt compelled to help them. What good am I to my patients if I cannot actually make them feel better? I then made it my life's ambition to research options available outside the "Western medicine box." I chose to investigate the voluminous, non-traditional, yet effective therapies found in the field of functional medicine instead of simply dismissing the symptoms plaguing my patients as associated with aging and offering them a huge hug and a strong sedative.

Some women transition through menopause without many symptoms. It is simply, "Wow, my period stopped! Oh well." If that is you, wonderful—but stick around because the latter part of this book (a few anti-aging secrets) is for you. On the flip side, many women are so significantly affected that managing through one day is literally impossible. Fortunately, this is extreme and not very common. However, most women experience symptoms that fall somewhere in the middle. They are significantly inconvenienced but not debilitated. If you do not fall in the middle, then more than likely, you have a girlfriend or two who does.

As you choose your holistic practitioner to help you through this season of your life, it is important to understand their credentials. My patients appreciate the fact that I have practiced gynecology for over 30 years and have focused primarily on hormone balancing and menopause wellness for the last 16 years. I read all the studies and keep abreast of the literature in both Western traditional medicine and regenerative holistic medicine. The wealth of knowledge I have obtained has allowed me to offer women a safe, effective, and convenient alternative to synthetic traditional hormones. Taking advantage of the benefits of these safe and effective modalities ensures a woman of "a certain age" can thrive and soar during the best years of her life. Contrary to popular belief, the best years are *after* 40!

Last time you checked, you were vibrant, vivacious, exuberant, and alive. Slowly, you became edgy, irritable, cranky, hot, and chubby. What happened to your woohoo? As a gynecologist, I have always focused on menopause wellness, specifically balancing the female hormones associated with menopause: estrogen, testosterone, and progesterone. So, I get it because I am trained and also because I am a woman who has gone through it. I now am that woman of "a certain age," and when the symptoms of perimenopause hit me, I needed a little help. Now, I am thriving, feeling, and looking younger and more vibrant than ever. I want to share *all* of my secrets about how to stay absolutely fabulous forever. I have even included a few other secrets from colleagues of mine in different fields.

This book will explain the changes you are experiencing and offer safe and effective options that allow you to exhilarate again. It is important to remember that menopause wellness does not preclude you from all of the other innovative and supportive therapies available for your total well-being. The first part of the book is the medical stuff—the need-to-know information about your perimenopause and menopause health. The second part? That is the fun part of life on the other side of "a certain age," from what happens in the bedroom to picking out the best clothes! The focus of my practice and this book is to explain how the bio-identical balancing of the female hormones in my patients has led them to a more fulfilling life, along with other need-to-know secrets that keep a woman *Absolutely Fabulous*!

For many years, so many patients, friends, and family—especially those amazing patients whose lives I have been honored to touch have emphatically stated to me, "You have to write a book!!" So here I am, and the great part is that this subject—that was once a hush-hush topic—is now being talked about more and more. I am not surprised that both perimenopause and menopause are all over the news. I'm even more excited that corporate companies are looking into how they can make their workplaces menopause friendly. It certainly is not because this is a trend but more so because women who have been suffering are not being quiet about it anymore. And they should not have to be hush-hush about it in order to make the next person (men) comfortable.

So many women and men have benefited from the life-enhancing therapies we offer in our wellness and anti-aging medical practice. Although this book is not going to be your one-stop shop, it will put you on the right track to understanding how effective bio-identical hormone balancing can be for you and, perhaps, a reason why you should give my office a call. Living *Absolutely Fabulous* does not mean that every day will be sunny and rainbows, it means that you should not suffer unnecessarily. If you are ready to learn how you can start or continue living your most fabulous life, regardless of your age, keep reading!

SECTION 1

BEHIND THE EXAM ROOM DOORS

CHAPTER

ONE

If you have experienced any of the following: covers off and on at night, unusually cranky, edgy, sweating the small stuff, fan in your purse, by your bed—or really a fan anywhere, then you are in good company. What about naked and wondering where your curves went? Cannot get that weight off, dead in bed? I am not done just yet...sex? Please, who has the energy or desire? What about if you can't remember what you were just googling or why you cannot sleep? And my all-time favorite—where is the bathroom because you gotta go? I have been there, and my patients have, too, so I know all about what you are either experiencing or have no interest in experiencing when it comes to perimenopause and menopause.

In the next few chapters, I am going to give you the need-to-know information about perimenopause, menopause, and bio-identical hormone balancing. It will also be intertwined with the stories of a few of my patients who went from miserable to fabulous. It is important for you to know that you are not alone, and you are most certainly not crazy.

Not only does bio-identical hormone balancing work for my patients, but these women had the same symptoms you might be having. They started where you are, miserable and wondering what in the world was going on with their bodies. For the average woman, perimenopause usually starts around the mid-forties when the hormone levels in a woman's body begin to wax and wane, paralleling their erratic production by the ovaries. Some months, a woman feels absolutely amazing, and other months, the symptoms of irritability and misery predominate her existence. The months when she is feeling edgy and anxious are consistent with significantly diminished hormone production by the ovaries. The predominant culprit responsible for these symptoms in a mid-forties woman is decreasing production of testosterone.

My patient, Janet, is the youngest of the bunch at 44. I was honored to deliver her now 18-year-old twins. Needless to say, I have known her for a long time. What I also know is that she has a fabulous relationship with her husband, their father, who she adores dearly. They raised their babies, were basking in their success, and were looking forward to being empty nesters as the twins were heading to their dream colleges and into the limitless world that awaited them.

One day, Janet admitted to me that she had lost her desire to have sex, her energy was lower than normal, she could not sleep, and she was gaining weight. Like many of us who live busy lives, it was easy for her to blame it on her long and exhausting days. However, when the energy and the sexual desire never seemed to come back, the red flags popped up, and so did a strong desire to understand what was happening with her body. Unlike Janet, her husband's sex drive was not waning, and he still had plenty of energy. So, to ignite the fire back into her marriage and figure out where her energy was going, she sought my professional help.

Sex may or may not seem like a big deal to some people. However, research has shown that low sexual satisfaction is linked to memory decline. Scientists have found that if you experience low sexual satisfaction (a typical menopause symptom), then you are at a higher risk for health problems that lead to cognitive decline[1]. Having more sex reduces stress and improves sleep and immunity. This sounds like something we all want unless you are just not in the mood and, worst of all, cannot figure out why you are not.

When a woman seeks answers from her Western-trained physician about her perimenopause and menopause symptoms, she is offered routine blood work, which evaluates her various systems and their functions. Many times, women do not know that they are in perimenopause to even bring it up to their doctor, so they go along with whatever the doctor wants to test. Obviously, there must be something major going on. The lab tests ordered usually include a check for anemia, kidney and liver function, electrolytes, diabetes, and, of course, the thyroid. They will also check the different female hormones. When all the results are within the Western lab's normal limits, the woman receives a call with a warm voice reassuring her that all her tests are normal. She then asks herself how her tests can be normal if she still feels pretty miserable.

---

[1] Penn State. (2023, May 30). Low sexual satisfaction linked to memory decline later in life. *ScienceDaily*. Retrieved June 5, 2024 from www.sciencedaily.com/releases/2023/05/230530125414.htm

Something is wrong. Something has to be wrong. She begs the question, "What about my irritability, anxiety, mood swings, weight gain, insomnia, and forgetfulness?" These symptoms herald perimenopause and are characteristics of the symptoms of declining testosterone production consistent with reaching the mid-forties. Perimenopause is often the last thing that a woman wants to consider— especially if she still has a cycle, even if it is not every month.

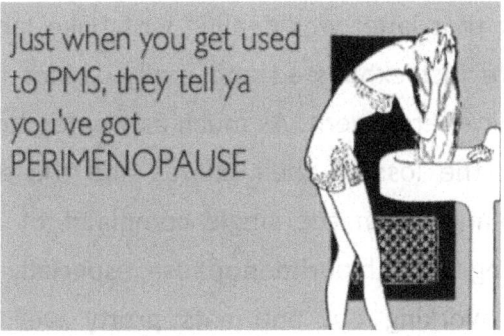

Most people and medical professionals are not familiar with how important testosterone is for women. Studies suggest testosterone has a direct effect on the brain receptors affecting memory, moods, and vitality. Women need testosterone, too, albeit a tiny tenth of what men require. However, that tiny tenth of testosterone is life-altering. Many of the symptoms of testosterone deficiency were simply accepted as unavoidable and untreatable.

When a woman sought answers from her traditional Western practitioners, they sadly departed their office visit with very few answers and even fewer solutions. Unfortunately, many women are often told to increase their activity and get more rest. As a kind gesture, the doctor may prescribe a mild sedative to help them relax and sleep.

This decrease in testosterone levels results in low energy, irritability, moodiness, difficulty sleeping, and weight gain. Everything that Janet was dealing with. Like Janet, many women are just exhausted and really cannot figure out where their energy went. As much as women love feeling energized, the loss of their curves and the associated weight gain is often the single complaint of a woman transitioning through perimenopause, especially when she has been working out and eats pretty well. Yet, her previously toned body is now welcoming the arrival of a muffin top.

Janet's symptoms were primarily consistent with testosterone deficiency. After balancing Janet with convenient subcutaneous bio-identical testosterone, she is "Girl on Fire" in her bedroom! "Her husband is happy" is the understatement of the year!! The kids better not drop by unannounced if they do not want to be embarrassed. To make things even better, her lost curves returned with her workout when she added weightlifting to strengthen and tone her muscles. She used to be intimidated by the machines in the gym, but after enlisting the guidance of a personal trainer, she has her workout routine perfected, and her body shows off the effort.

CHAPTER
TWO

Women do not wake up one day all of a sudden in menopause. Perimenopause usually happens first. Whether a woman is really noticing the changes in her body or not during that time, it is what happens as her body transitions to menopause. Perimenopause and menopause are heralded by missing periods, which ultimately cease. Well, to be real—she probably does not really miss her period. However, since her ovaries are not cycling, the absence of the cycle causes estrogen production to decrease, and she begins the misery of hot flashes and night sweats. I can assure you that the excitement of her not getting her menses is not long-lasting.

Menopause is a discreet point in time defined by the absence of a cycle for one year. The word menopause, by definition, simply means no more periods—period. Therefore, a woman is either in her reproductive years with cyclic bleeding or skipping periods (perimenopause) until she reaches the point where her periods have ceased, and she is in the menopause era of her life—for the rest of her life. So, if a woman starts to bleed well after that time, something else is going on and she should be immediately evaluated.

With menopause, the symptoms a woman experienced during perimenopause are often more intense and persistent—the joys of being a woman. Because of that, when a woman refers to "menopause," she is usually referring to the irritating and often disabling symptoms associated with that time in her life. In most cases, she is only bringing it up because she is having symptoms that are emotionally and physically debilitating and dramatically interfering with her productivity and existence.

The average age span of the onset of menopause is between 47 to 51 years. However, the symptoms of perimenopause can begin as early as the thirties and extend throughout the remainder of your life. Fortunately for many women, the debilitating symptoms of early menopause often ease as a woman ages. The hot flashes and night sweats that typically begin around age 47 to 51 start to decrease and become manageable as a woman transitions to her mid to late fifties and then gradually diminish during the 60s. Something physiologically changes around age 80. Ask any woman you know in their 80s and 90s—they always have a little something covering their arms and a little something covering their head to protect them from the breeze when they go outside.

Our next miserable to fabulous patient, Sharon (62), a very successful investment banker, can probably write a book about hot flashes and night sweats. Her symptoms were affecting every aspect of her existence to the point where her presentations at work were marred by dripping sweats and forgetfulness. She was edgy, irritable, irrational, and, most of all, embarrassed. When she first sought my care, all I had to offer her was the highest doses of synthetic estrogen available, and she still did not attain any resolution of her debilitating symptoms. One night, she called me exasperated and said she had walked into her backyard and into her pool. The problem was that it was a cold October evening, and the pool was not heated. She was so desperate that she chose an arctic plunge for relief. I shiver just thinking about it. As her trusted physician, I felt compelled to help her. Her life depended on her sharp and productive mind. Her job depended on it, especially since she was losing allies and support at work because her colleagues were now referring to her as "cranky Sharon!"

Society is not forgiving towards women when they reach "a certain age." Our bodies are doing what they are made to do as we age and slow down the production of certain hormones. Unfortunately, Sharon is not the only one whose work performance is at risk when perimenopause and menopause start to set in. A British study found that one-third of women ages 50 to 64 reported moderate to severe difficulties coping at work because of menopausal symptoms[2].

I am sure, at this point, you are probably wondering why you must have these symptoms to begin with. After dealing with your menses and its associated PMS symptoms for decades, it would be much easier if your period just left quietly without making a fuss. The simple response is that the symptoms of perimenopause and menopause are associated with diminished hormone production. These hormones, which are produced by the endocrine glands,

---

[2] Otterman, S., & Paskova, Y. (2023, May 22). A Movement to Make Workplaces "Menopause Friendly." *The New York Times*.
https://www.nytimes.com/2023/05/22/nyregion/menopause-women-work.html

are integral to the delicate, intricate mechanics of all the processes going on in our bodies. This is how our body communicates and transmits important messages to ensure balance. When balanced and producing adequate hormones, the endocrine systems function like a well-oiled and calibrated machine. Specifically, we experience a sense of overall well-being. Hormone balancing is important to a woman's immunity, mood, energy levels, libido, and the inner workings of her cardiac and neuromuscular systems.

When we think about what hormones are important to the physiological functioning of the body, we can categorize them as primary or secondary. The thyroid and pancreas are vital to optimal living and are considered primary endocrine organs. Diabetes and hypothyroidism are the names of the diseases that result from an inadequately functioning pancreas and thyroid, respectively. However, deciding not to balance and support these organs when they are insufficient would result in disability and, ultimately, death. Contrarily, the hormones produced in the ovaries and adrenals—estrogen, testosterone, and progesterone—are considered secondary hormones. As secondary hormones, a woman's health will not be compromised when they are diminished. However, when these hormones are balanced, a woman lives a fuller, more fabulous existence. This is why it is important for women to know they do not have to just "live with it" and continue to be inconvenienced. Since perimenopause and menopause are consistent with decreased ovarian and adrenal production of these hormones, it is easy to now understand why the symptoms a woman experiences during this time are symptoms associated primarily with waning estrogen and testosterone levels.

CHAPTER

THREE

During menopause, estrogen production is significantly decreased and often negligible to absent. Estrogen receptors are predominantly in the vaginal tissue, the breast, the bones, skin, and brain. Because of the location of estrogen receptors in these strategic areas, a woman's body is perky, lush, vibrant, and alive during her reproductive years when estrogen is plentiful. At the time of menopause, the symptoms of estrogen deficiency are most visibly exhibited in these areas. With estrogen hormone balancing, a woman experiences relief from those unbearable and unpredictable hot flashes and night sweats. Her hair and makeup stay perfect, her clothes fit without that dribble of sweat, *and* the vaginal dryness and painful sex that she may have been experiencing decreases tremendously. The confidence that returns to her life is empowering and exhilarating.

Plain and simply stated, men eagerly desire women who want to have sex with them! However, when it hurts to do it, it is hard to be interested. In many women, estrogen and testosterone balancing, just like a genie's magic wand, has often returned that desire with the first bio-identical hormone insertion procedure. We have proudly restored pleasure in the bedroom and included the added benefits of energy, memory, focus, balanced mood, great sleep, weight loss, and the return of those curves you missed.

The endocrine organs (pancreas, adrenals, ovaries, thyroid) were designed to supply all of the intricate physiological workings of a woman's body throughout her reproductive years. Prior to the twentieth century, a woman's life expectancy was about fifty years. Meaning women died soon after their reproductive years ended. With the technological advances in science and the development of antibiotics to treat previously fatal infections, women not only began to live beyond the reproductive years but twice as long. Conversely, the endocrine organs were not equipped to adapt to enhanced longevity and optimally sustain a woman through her advancing years. A woman's life expectancy increased, yet her vital endocrine organs did not increase their productivity to parallel these phenomena. Now, women experiencing symptoms consistent with the decrease in the production of hormones from the endocrine organs can seek early medical intervention and supplementation.

Women aged 40 to 45 often experience the symptoms of testosterone's gradual decline, and women aged 47 to 55 are experiencing the added and often dramatic symptoms of sudden estrogen deficiency. Suddenly and dramatically, the hormones have disappeared. Almost like yesterday, a woman's hormones were flourishing, and then they were whisked away overnight.

There are ample articles within the curriculum of integrative or regenerative medicine addressing hormone imbalance in general and testosterone imbalance in particular. Because integrative medicine and bio-identical hormone balancing is a relatively new curriculum and has only recently been taught in medical school, many practicing physicians are not aware of the information and the solutions they offer.

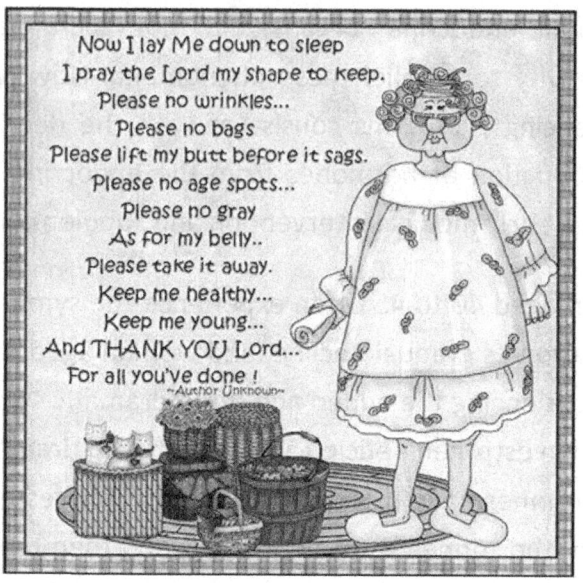

Now I lay Me down to sleep
I pray the Lord my shape to keep.
Please no wrinkles...
Please no bags
Please lift my butt before it sags.
Please no age spots...
Please no gray
As for my belly..
Please take it away.
Keep me healthy...
Keep me young...
And THANK YOU Lord...
For all you've done !
~Author Unknown~

Each woman's experience is as individual as she is. Some women find relief using numerous herbs and supplements available in reputable holistic health stores. Others add the addition of yoga and other mindful activities coupled with self-care, and they can transition uneventfully through perimenopause and menopause. Then, there are the women who need a lot more assistance to balance their hormones. Not much of anything they have tried has worked.

Today's woman refuses to accept anything less than the vitality and exuberant spirit, as well as the toned, luscious look of Jennifer Lopez and Halle Berry. They do not want the frump of Blanche from Golden Girls. JLo and Halle are the *new* 50. If not the body exactly, a woman wants confidence. The desire for vitality parallels with a woman's ascent into decision-making positions in the job market. She wants to continue to own and lead it and be the ultimate "boss babe." She wants to command the room with her beautiful, exuberant brilliance. Yes, she wants and can have it all with the right support. She also wants to own her sex life and not be afraid of it. As I have mentioned before, sexuality and intimacy are essential elements for quality of life across the board[3]. Bio-identical hormone supplementation of the missing secondary hormones allows a woman's body and mind to be supported and nourished as she continues to ascend and soar in her new era of menopause.

---

[3] Society, T. N. A. M. (2022, January 19). *The link among resilience, sexual function, and quality of life in menopausal women.* Medicalxpress.com.
https://medicalxpress.com/news/2022-01-link-resilience-sexual-function-quality.html

FOUR

Many women can pinpoint the day or the event when they first experienced their first hot flash. Sarah told me she was attending a formal event when her symptoms started. Her hair, makeup, and dress were flawless. She was fabulous. She was standing on the dance floor, and all of a sudden, she felt dribbles of sweat run down the inside of her thighs, pooling down to her ankles. It was so bad that she actually thought she was going to make a puddle on the floor. All she wanted to do was get under a brisk shower of ice-cold water. Hair and makeup? Forget it. Her hot dress became a fiery furnace.

She hurried into the ladies' room dripping and begged for help from the obviously experienced inhabitants. Imbued with empathy, they advised her to run her wrists under cold water and suggested she refrain from alcohol and caffeine and discretely place her inner wrists around a glass of ice if the hot flash returned. She made it through the evening and hurried to her GYN's office as soon as she could. Whew! She was offered what she knew to be available and effective (the one-size-fits-all synthetic options) to relieve the hot flashes. The Premarin was effective, and the Prometrium helped her sleep, but what about the other nagging symptoms that had started? She was experiencing irritability and was so mean and edgy. Valium and Xanax were offered, and she adamantly refused.

Synthetic hormones were once the only option, with Premarin leading the race for the go-to option. Every pharmaceutical company desired to be the manufacturer of the next best thing. These synthetic hormones merely suppress the symptoms associated with perimenopause and menopause but do nothing to support the underlying cause of what is really occurring. Endocrine organ insufficiency and depletion are the issues, and the endocrine organ must be replenished to achieve optimal wellness. Simply suppressing the associated symptoms of hormone deficiency is not the holistic answer.

Consider a torn ACL ligament in the knee. Taking synthetic hormones to offer relief from the symptoms of menopause can be compared to taking ibuprofen to relieve the pain and swelling caused by a torn ACL, yet doing nothing to support or heal the damaged ligament so the knee can function again. The pain and swelling may be relieved for a while, but the knee does not function *because* the ligament is torn. Just like ibuprofen cannot heal a torn ACL, synthetic hormones cannot supply the vital yet declining production of the endocrine hormones by their respective glands.

As the name suggests, synthetic hormones are artificially made, and they may offer a temporary resolution of symptoms, but they don't support the root cause of hormone deficiency because they are made from artificial ingredients in a laboratory of chemists. Bio-identical hormones supplement the deficient endocrine gland and the receptors located in the body. Synthetic hormones may be somewhat similar to the hormones the endocrine organs produce, but somewhat similar is not enough. The reality is, when it comes to our hormones, unless it is exact, it does not work exactly. Since the body does not recognize these synthetic hormones as its own, untoward severe and often fatal side effects can be associated. The untoward side effects that are heralded in the news are associated with synthetic hormones *only*. Since no delineation has been made, the listening public believes "hormones are hormones." This is far from the truth, and in order to make the best decision for your health, you need to be armed with facts.

The facts we know are that synthetic hormone usage can be associated with an increased risk of female cancers, especially of the breast. In the infamous Women's Health Initiative study that came out in 2002, synthetic hormones were found to increase the risk of breast cancer. Specifically, invasive breast cancer findings were significant enough that the study had to be abruptly halted because patients were being harmed. The culprits studied in this report were Premarin (the estrogen) and Provera (the progesterone). Both of these hormones are synthetic, and Provera is archaic. The Premarin-only arm of the study was allowed to continue because there was no increase in breast cancer in these participating women. This evidence suggested estrogen alone was perhaps not the culprit. In addition to the study, Premarin was no longer prescribed when concerns arose after women became aware of the origin of Premarin, horse urine. Animal activists set off that alarm.

With concerns of patient safety and, of course, liability, physicians abruptly stopped offering women synthetic hormones and insisted they not use ANY hormones because of the increased risk of breast cancer. Since a woman's prescription for her estrogen was not renewed by her physician, she then asked the question, "What now? What can I take that will reduce my symptoms and be safe for me?" Her physician responded most often with a reluctant shrug. Women were left to suffer or seek other options as their Western-trained physicians offered very little guidance, support, or encouragement. Women were offered potentially addictive sedatives with serious side effects or nothing at all. Neither was acceptable to many women who knew they could not and would not just grin and bear it. Being sedated or just miserable with drippy clothes, matted hair, and makeup was not an option. It is impossible to maximize a woman's potential when her existence is punctuated by these symptoms, and a woman should not have to simply accept the uncomfortable and often embarrassing symptoms of hormone imbalance. Today's woman demands more. They are on boards, they facilitate workshops and presentations, and they travel more extensively than their mothers and grandmothers.

Some women turn to supplements to find relief. When the sleepless nights accompanied by hot flashes begin, a woman may first go to her computer to research and then head to her nearest supplement store of choice to pick up the recommended options. Black Cohosh is the go-to supplement because it relieves hot flashes and night sweats, as well as irritability and mood swings. For many women, this is all they need.

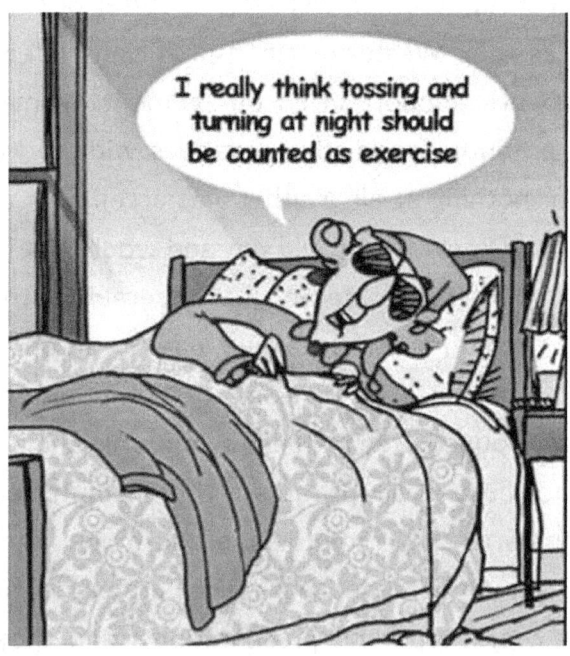

A restful and peaceful night's sleep free from night sweats is the result for many after consuming this supplement. Soy is another supplement that is similar to estrogen. Therefore, it may reduce the symptoms of hot flashes and night sweats. Dong Quai is a contribution from Asian herbal practitioners as it is also known to relieve hot flashes and night sweats. Since DHEA is a precursor of estrogen and testosterone, many use this supplement instead of taking estrogen and testosterone. If you are of the 15% feeling good after consuming these supplements, the rest of this section is for those in the 85th percentile.

Remember Janet, my patient with twins and the doting husband? Well, luckily for her, she stumbled across and started researching bio-identical hormone balancing as a possible option prior to her gynecologist discontinuing her synthetic hormones after the WHI study. She didn't want to be in a position where she was out of options if she was told she could no longer take the synthetic hormone that she depended on. Unfortunately, this was the experience of the majority of women. Doctors were basically telling suffering women that they had to find a way to live with their symptoms because a lot of the synthetic hormones were no longer prescribed. After the WHI study dimmed the light on hormone replacement therapy, women felt neglected and abandoned by the same providers who had been their support through their reproductive years.

Fortunately for my patients, they were already receiving plant-based bio-identical hormones as a long-term resolution of the present urgent and debilitating symptoms associated with menopause.

FIVE

Bio-identical hormones, in contrast to synthetic hormones, are plant-based and replenish the deficient endocrine organs. Since they are natural plant-based supplements made from yam, bio-identical hormones do not increase a woman's risk of breast cancer. It is important to note that bio-identical hormones do not protect the breast from cancer because the causes of breast cancer are multifactorial. In balancing, caution is and should always be to offer a woman only enough bio-identical estrogen to diminish her hot flashes, protect her bones, and keep her skin soft and supple. The combination of estrogen and vaginal moisturizers like vitamin E oil keeps the vagina ripe, succulent, and ready. A small dose of estrogen, in addition to testosterone, strengthens and sustains the bones, preventing osteoporosis. If a woman with thin bones slips and falls, this could result in a hip fracture and subsequent immobilization as she is prescribed bed rest for the bones to fuse. This immobilization could trigger a serious infection or a pulmonary embolism, resulting in death. Because of the life-sustaining importance of the prevention of osteoporosis, the long-term benefits of bio-identical hormone balancing should be considered.

Within the specialty of integrative/regenerative medicine lies the vast knowledge of bio-identical hormones. Bio-identical hormones are formulated by licensed compounding pharmacists in accredited and regulated sterile labs. These specialized compounded hormones are plant-based and are prepared to the exact specifications of the hormones that the endocrine organs in the body produce. Because of this exactness, bio-identical compounded hormones support and replenish the body exactly as if this hormone were made in the endocrine organ in the body. Every woman is different, and so is their dosage of hormone supplements. Bio-identical hormones can be taken orally, topically, or in the form of a pellet.

Although there are many bio-identical options available, after years of research evaluating the different options, our office specializes in bio-identical hormones using the subcutaneous pellets delivery system. Pellets are newer to the U.S. market, but European women have been using pellets since the early 1900s. However, even women who are using or are open to using bio-identical hormones may not automatically want pellets because of a lack of information. This is our method of choice because of its convenience and health benefits. A patient visits us about every four months for the insertion of fresh hormone pellets.

When hormones are introduced into the body, it is important that they are presented in the safest and most effective form. Estradiol is the most significant and effective estrogen for hormone balancing, yet when ingested, it is changed in the liver to a less active form known as estrone. The processing of estradiol by the liver may also release proteins that increase the risk of blood clots in the legs, which could migrate to the lungs. When choosing your method of delivery of hormones, it is a healthier option to bypass the liver because you present a purer, more effective product to your bloodstream and to the body's awaiting depleted receptors. Creams and patches afford the same benefits, yet the absorption can be inconsistent and unpredictable. Our skin is meant to protect us. Thus, it is the most difficult organ to permeate.

Although creams are a widely used option, they have to be applied daily. This can often be a cumbersome ask for many women, and for many women, this is simply too burdensome.

Using the subcutaneous insertion, we can administer pellets under the skin directly into the subcutaneous layer (think adipose tissue) to be absorbed by the bloodstream, which delivers the hormone to the depleted receptors. We insert it in the upper hip area of the back at the top of the thong line. So, it is your little secret. With this direct method, we can give our patients the lowest dosage of hormones to achieve the desired result. Typically, they will start to feel better within a few days to a week after receiving the insertion. Also, utilizing the subcutaneous method of delivery bypasses the stomach and the liver. This is an important feature because any medicine that enters the stomach has to be coated to prevent destruction by acidic gastric juices. In addition, many medicines are changed to a less-than-desirable form when they pass through the liver. Bypassing both the stomach and liver ensures the pure bio-identical hormone is the product that is delivered to the receptors in the body.

We feel pellets are a superior choice because they are small, and inserting them is almost pain-free. They bypass the liver, offer predictable absorption of the hormones in your body, and are convenient. I am not discrediting creams, patches, or any other option. When patients request these alternatives, our compounding pharmacy is ready to comply. However, visiting your provider every four months for pellet insertion compared with daily dosing is extremely attractive to someone who wants to get back to their fabulous life with little inconvenience.

I will add that initially our patient Janet tried testosterone cream but did not notice appreciable results, and any results she did see were not consistent. Ultimately, she chose subcutaneous pellet insertion of bio-identical testosterone to ensure predictable, carefree, and fabulous results. She returns every four months for her fresh testosterone pellet re-boost. As she approaches 50, she may experience hot flashes and night sweats, but we have that under control as well. After lab work and another consultation, estrogen and progesterone can be added to her formulation to support this deficiency. With plant-based bio-identical balancing, the goal is to supplement the endocrine organs so they can safely and effectively produce wonderful healing and regenerative hormones for a woman as they did in her 30s and early 40s.

When Sharon, the 62-year-old CEO, came into my office, her symptoms and laboratory values confirmed a significant deficiency in both estrogen and testosterone. Her schedule did not allow daily hormone dosing because she was always flying off somewhere and would certainly miss the dosing schedule or leave the hormones at home. When she was offered the subcutaneous insertion of bio-identical hormones in the form of pellets, she grasped the opportunity to feel fabulous again with a carefree method of administration. Nothing to pack and nothing to remember to take. We balanced her hormones with bio-identical estrogen and testosterone pellets placed painlessly under her skin and added progesterone oral supplementation to support and protect her uterus from overstimulation by the estrogen.

We primarily offer progesterone therapy using the oral route, as this method of administration allows us to easily tailor the dosing for the patient. It was a necessary additive because it also ensured patients like Sharon get a full night of much needed sleep. Sharon awakens every morning productive and profitable as she leads her successful financial company. She can sense it when her hormones are waning, and she promised herself never to spend one miserable moment unbalanced. Her quarterly appointment for hormone balancing is inked in her calendar.

The transition from perimenopause into menopause should be anticipated with exuberant enthusiasm. After the immediate symptoms associated with menopause are resolved, a woman's focus should be directed toward protecting her body as she ages. The longevity and anti-aging benefits of hormone balancing are as important as the immediate relief of symptoms of perimenopause.

I would be remiss if I didn't mention that the work I do in my office is not always well received by traditional Western physicians. Even with all the proof of how well the pellets work and how well the body receives them. Many times, when a patient returns to her primary care physician to tell them how wonderful she is feeling after starting hormone balancing therapy with me, she becomes the recipient of words like, "Bio-Identical...that is a bunch of nonsense. There is no value to that," or they might tell her, "A bunch of doctors will try to sell you a bunch of junk!" A colleague of mine once suggested to me that when doctors are not up on something, they are down on it. I know their responses are a lack of knowledge because I used to be one of them. However, what grinds my gears is when my patients are told that what we give them is not FDA-approved or it is not real medicine.

That is simply not true. As I mentioned before, everything inside of our pellets is created in an accredited and regulated compounding pharmacy by licensed pharmacists, and the ingredients are FDA-approved—every single one of them. Where most people get hung up on is the method in which these are delivered. Delivery by pellets is "not" approved, and honestly, that is unimportant in this situation.

CHAPTER

SIX

I know that most of this information can be scary, and when given the option and knowledge, what woman would willingly choose to take something that has such a high risk of breast cancer? The WHI study may have been problematic for physicians who were prescribing synthetic hormones very often, but it was extremely impactful for women like my client Phyllis (68), who has a family history of breast cancer. Although Phyllis was no longer experiencing hot flashes, she was concerned because the results of her recent bone density scan showed osteopenia, an early sign of decreased bone density. At age 87, her mom had been diagnosed with osteoporosis, significantly decreased bone tissue, and died from the complications of a hip fracture sustained after a slip and fall. The hip fracture was caused by her mom's fragile, thin bones, and her mom ultimately succumbed to the consequences of immobilization necessary to mend the fracture. When Phyllis shared her mom's history with her internist, her physician suggested she start bone-strengthening medications immediately and offered her the latest and greatest. When the side effects were reviewed with her, Phyllis felt there must be other options that could strengthen her bones yet not increase her chances of developing breast cancer. Phyllis wanted a brighter *rest* of her life than her mom and aunt (who suffered from dementia), and she wanted more natural and individual options than those offered by her traditional Western practitioners.

Since Phyllis was concerned about her strong family history of breast cancer and osteoporosis, we wanted to give her complete control over her dosing of bio-identical estrogen. We, therefore, initiated her estrogen in the form of a bio-identical transdermal cream and progressed to the bio-identical patch as she sought more relief from flashes and support for her bones. Calcium and vitamin D were added to augment her regimen further. Using these self-administered dosing options, Phyllis was able to achieve the bone, bladder, and vaginal support she deserved. The addition of bio-identical testosterone in the form of the convenient sub-dermal pellet was given for her brain support, especially her memory, and the testosterone further strengthened her bones. As an added bonus, she received the PRP vaginal rejuvenation—which I'll discuss more in a later chapter—to restore her bladder support. Phyllis is strong, balanced, and dry—no more pee pads for her. Most importantly, her breast cancer fears are alleviated. A follow-up bone density scan confirmed the effectiveness of estrogen supplementation.

Tailored and individualized relief of the debilitating symptoms of hormone deficiency is available for all women who desire an extraordinary existence. Since menopause, or the time in a woman's life when she no longer menstruates, is for the duration of her life, she may experience profound lifelong consequences of hormone imbalance and depletion. As a woman contemplates long-term bio-identical hormone balancing, she should consider the benefits of this being a life-long treatment.

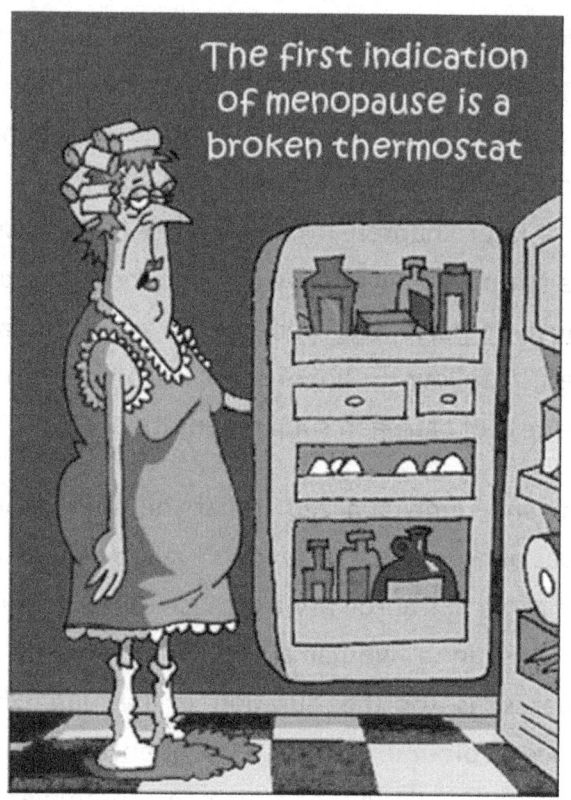

The known long-term benefits of bio-identical hormone balancing are ensuring keen brain function with the prevention of Alzheimer's and dementia. Bio-identical hormone balancing, complemented with weight-bearing exercise, vitamin D, and calcium, supports a strong, solid bone matrix. Long-term hormone balancing also ensures a strong, healthy heart and imparts a supported bladder and a vibrant vagina. We prepare financially for our latter years. It is time that we prepare our body, mind, and spirit for optimum wellness and well-being.

CHAPTER

SEVEN

It's not a secret or an unknown fact anymore that the symptoms of perimenopause and menopause affect a woman's effectiveness and bottom line—i.e., her money! When you wake up irritable, edgy, and with brain fog, your productivity is diminished. When your productivity is diminished, your bottom line is affected. We must correlate balanced hormones with the profit of your enterprise. This hasn't been talked about until recently—especially in the media. The following are symptoms associated with the hormone deficiencies accompanying perimenopause and menopause that directly diminish your bottom line.

When a woman experiences a loss of clarity and energy, she has less focus, and her production and creativity are low. This results in her missing deadlines and goals. It impacts her payroll because she may be absent using sick days or have a short-term disability. If she works for herself or another company, her low creativity affects her decision-making and what she brings to the table. Not only does this impact her but also those she works with, and it could cause a financial burden on the company as a whole.

It may sound extreme, but imagine you own a very successful company, and Bobbi is your top person who reports directly to your CFO. If your CFO were absent, she could do their job. Bobbi is a numbers guru and the go-to person for perfection and ingenuity. As soon as she turned the BIG 5-0, it seemed like hot flashes started to melt her during the day, extend through the night, and interrupt her rest. Her mornings feel like she hasn't rested at all, and recovery is impossible. She had always been a boss in the boardroom, but now she has been late for meetings and cannot figure out why she does not know why she's late. Her short-term lack of prioritization translates into decreased productivity, profits, and the bottom line for herself and your company. Eventually, you are forced to hire a temp, Marina, to cover Bobbi when she requests PTO. There is a business cost of temps and a cost to the productivity with the lag associated with onboarding someone to do Bobbi's job—add this to the non-monetary cost of Bobbi's absence from her projects.

Either way you put it, menopause costs, and most of the time, the woman experiencing it pays the higher price. The Mayo Clinic reported that menopause costs American women an estimated $1.8 billion in lost working time a year[4]. Some women take a few days off here and there, but there is a small percentage of women who quit their jobs altogether because their symptoms are so debilitating. They think it is better to resign than to be fired due to their excessive absences or not being able to perform their duties when they are at work. Menopause can strike at any time, but most women experience it when they are at the top of their careers. Although it is recommended that women see doctors who specialize in menopause to get their symptoms managed, companies have a role to play as well.

Many companies have either been fiscally impacted or saw that they could lose money if their bottom line was impacted by a woman who was experiencing the

---

[4] Gupta, A. H. (2023, April 28). Study Shows the Staggering Cost of Menopause for Women in the Work Force. *The New York Times.* https://www.nytimes.com/2023/04/28/well/live/menopause-symptoms-work-women.html#:~:text=Some%20are%20taking%20sick%20days

symptoms associated with perimenopause and menopause. Human Resources are beginning to develop a sensitivity and, therefore, support women experiencing reproductive issues like infertility and pre and post-natal complications. It is time to also recognize the need for perimenopause and menopause support. In all honesty, the best place to start is education. Like everything else, when a person (regardless of gender) is educated on a topic, they can then move and make changes accordingly. Menopause does not have to be a taboo topic, and the women experiencing it do not have to be labeled as "cranky," "moody," or "irritable." Unfortunately, because it is a hush-hush topic, there is fear around what companies might think of a woman doing her job as she ages. They may say the older she gets, the harder work becomes for her[5].

Here's something else that menopause is costing women— their mental health. I have heard my patients tell me repeatedly that they feel like they might be slightly losing it because they cannot find relief and do not know what the problem is. Some women find themselves seeing their therapist a lot more frequently. Other women are asking

---

[5] Otterman, S., & Paskova, Y. (2023, May 22). A Movement to Make Workplaces "Menopause Friendly." *The New York Times*.

their doctors to prescribe sedatives to help them relax and sleep or antidepressants so they can get through their days better. Although these may seem like really appropriate therapy options for younger women, it is almost always not the solution for a woman in perimenopause or menopause. Our mental health is most often related to our balanced hormones during the mid-forties and beyond. When a woman is balanced hormonally, she has improved mental acuity.

There are many fears around the conversation of menopause, and some of them start in our homes. We saw our mothers and our grandmothers suffer. Unless we see a knowledgeable professional, we may end up with a lot of unanswered questions. Regardless, managing your menopause symptoms to be the best version of yourself does not start with the media or your job, and it does not start with the people around you. It starts with you. You must be the one to advocate for yourself with the information you have been given and refuse to experience what generations before you experienced. Nothing works overnight, but treatment works fairly quickly. Whether you need this information today—or in the future, the decision to manage your hormones and live an absolutely fabulous life is entirely up to you.

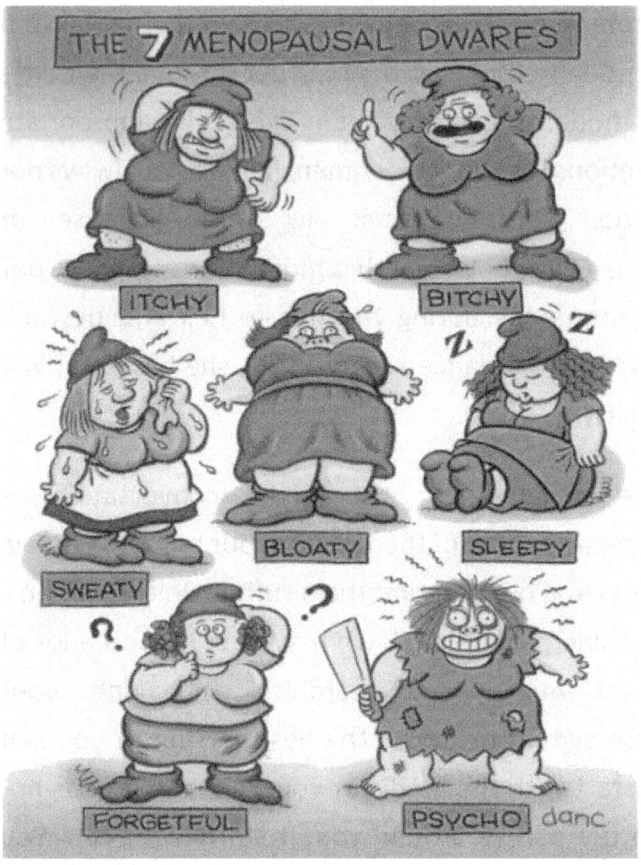

EIGHT

Hot flashes and mood changes are not the only things that women have to worry about when menopause starts. Our vagina starts to act its age, and we may experience the "gotta goes" or we "piddle when we giggle." Many women wear a pee pad when they go to Zumba class, or they think twice about tennis and pickleball. For some women, it has been happening well before they reach perimenopause. If you have delivered kids and have a sexual partner, then this is probably you. Incontinence? No, that's grandma in the nursing home who wears those diapers. Women in their perimenopause and menopause age "peez when they sneeze," but we are not incontinent. What we are experiencing is decreased bladder control caused by a combination of the decreased estrogen in the receptors around the urethra that support the neck of the bladder and the pelvic floor weakness caused by the delivery of your kids.

In addition to our estrogen hormone balancing, we offer our signature procedure, which is called the LADYLYFT. Yes, the LADYLYFT because she needs a spa day, too. You have asked a lot of her. Babies and years of happy bedroom time have made her more than deserving. What exactly is the LADYLYFT? Well, the name you would Google is called the O-shot, but the LADYLIFT is our signature name. For this procedure, we use platelet-rich plasma (PRP), which is the mechanism the body uses to heal and regenerate its own tissues. Think of it this way: if you cut yourself as a kid, the body healed by regenerating its own tissue. So, how do we get the PRP? We simply draw a blood sample as if you were getting labs for cholesterol, and we get rid of the red blood cells because we don't need them. What's left is what we call liquid gold—platelet-rich plasma. Once it is activated, it can be inserted into any tissue in the body, and the cells are regenerated.

If you ask any athlete, they have probably had a PRP injection in the knee for complete healing and support of the ligaments and the joints. It is often used as an adjunct to therapy or surgery or just in place of surgery for an injured meniscus. Orthopedics has been using it forever.

Many women have received PRP micro-needling in the face to regenerate and rejuvenate the facial skin and make it soft and supple like it used to be. It also rejuvenates and regenerates the facial skin to recover it from years of sun damage and decreasing estrogen. We use the same PRP, with its natural regenerative properties, in your vaginal area to regenerate and rejuvenate the vagina and support the urethra.

When a woman visits our office for the procedure, an anesthesia cream is liberally applied under the urethra and along the labia (lips of the vagina). As the anesthesia is absorbed, her blood is drawn and separated, and the PRP is prepared. After activation, a small amount is inserted under the urethra into the bladder neck. This is the area that supports the bladder and offers bladder control. Bladder support is improved by 80% and also decreases the "gotta goes" by 80%. Since this is also where your G-spot is, you get this added treat of G-spot enhancement and the pleasure it brings.

Women seek our signature LADYLYFT procedure to improve their bladder support and control. While performing this procedure, we can also reverse the effects of time and strategically place additional PRP to plump up the vaginal lips (vulva). Can you imagine the confidence you will have knowing you have bladder control and how pretty "down there" is? You are ready for your close-up and leave-the-lights-on kind of sex!!

My miserable to fabulous patient, Bobbi, is also newly divorced, available, and very desirous of dating. She often emphatically states that 48 was her best age, and she would have been happy to stay right there. Thank you very much! Yes, Bobbi will do any and everything to look and feel 48 for as long as she can. Along with her experiences with hot flashes, night sweats, difficulty sleeping, and being easily irritated, her two real issues are the loss of her curves, and she "piddles when she giggles." She came into my office wanting and needing to have better control over her life and her bladder. I recommended she receive testosterone hormone balancing in the form of pellets to maintain the strength and endurance of her muscles and bones, and a minimal dosage of bio-identical estrogen pellets was added to diminish her hot flashes and improve her vaginal support. To make her the happiest, she also received our vaginal rejuvenation procedure, the LADYLYFT, to regenerate the supportive muscles associated with bladder support and to vivify the vagina. Her labial lips are plumped, her clitoris enlivened, her bladder is supported, and her vagina is refreshed. Bobbi is now soaring exuberantly, and her vaginal area is vibrantly alive.

SECTION 2
LADIES NIGHT

CHAPTER

NINE

MOVE YOUR BODY

Loving and caring for your body needs to be at the top of your to-do list. Before you work on your relationship with others, you should work on your relationship with yourself to ensure you are doing your part to be in great health. It is important to love yourself better than anyone else can. Self-love is not about having it all together or meeting impossible standards. It is about embracing every part of who you are, including flaws and all. It is about acknowledging your worthiness, just as you are, and treating yourself with the kindness and compassion you deserve. Even if you are not the type to take a bunch of vitamins, squeezing in physical movement a few times a week will do wonders for your body—and yes, sex is included in that.

As you know, your body changes physically with age, and it probably has not maintained its youthful agility. It is still important to continue some physical activity. It is even encouraged to have a fitness routine that is realistic and manageable for the life you live—not the life you wish you lived. The flexibility of your joints and the strength of your muscles and bones is important for your longevity. Preparing your body for its peak performance in your latter years begins with baby steps now.

A great start is also increasing the distance and pace when walking. Water aerobics and dance classes are a fun way to connect with friends while having a good workout. Doing this 30 minutes a day can do wonders for your weight and fitness levels. Most women do not exercise daily, so adding fun and fit classes can do wonders for your flexibility and weight. Fun aerobics activities also benefit you by decreasing the symptoms of menopause. They can lift your mood, improve your sleep, and decrease your anxiety. Many times, women have symptoms of feeling extra fatigued, even if their hormones are balanced, so they reach for that extra cup of joe. Aerobic activities are a great way to get an extra pick-me-up to finish or start your day strong. In previous chapters, we discussed the increased risk of osteoporosis for some women. Aerobic exercises actually improve lower body strength and balance, and these factors will help keep you more agile and stable.

Walking can both lower your risk of breast cancer and reduce the risk of heart disease by 30%. This alone is a huge reason to get up and get out. When thinking about walking, it doesn't always have to be walking around your neighborhood or on the treadmill. Any walk counts. You can walk around the mall or take a walking tour of your city. A lot of cities have walking and hiking trails, and depending on where you live, there are probably tons of activities and parks to go to. A quick Google search can tell you where to start. You can also try dancing, golf, pickleball, and running workouts to support your cardiovascular health.

You don't have to spend hours and hours at the gym and using all the machines they have to offer. You can take a class or two a week. Gyms typically offer a variety of daily fitness classes for different fitness levels, including aerobics, yoga, Zumba, ballet, step, barre, and swimming classes. You may even find that your local gym or YMCA partners with SilverSneakers—a fitness program for individuals 65 and older. If you prefer not to go to the gym, you can download their app and take classes at home. I will add that the benefit of going to the class is having the instructor readily available in the room to motivate you and assist you with proper posture to avoid injury.

You may not be looking for new friends, but taking these classes in person brings a level of socialization with them. Everyone is there for the same thing, to get or stay in shape. It's much more fun to work out with a group of people than to go at it alone all the time. The social aspect is an added benefit that you won't be able to get if you do all your exercising at home and by yourself—even if it is tempting. After you are done working out, some luxurious gyms have a wet room area in the locker room so you can reward yourself for your hard work.

If and when you decide to increase the types of exercises you do, strength exercises will help build and maintain muscle mass, some of which may have been lost during the onset of perimenopause. The different types include bodyweight exercises such as squats, planks, or a manageable version of push-ups. The best part about bodyweight exercises is that they do not require a trip to the gym or a subscription to any fitness site. They can be done anywhere you can carve out space and time. Perfect for the individual who is constantly on the go with the demands of an active life or one who does not want to be bothered with a gym membership.

Lifting weights is also great for your overall health. Of course, the recommendation is to start off with a small weight and, over time, gradually increase the amount you can lift. Other activities like hiking, kayaking, and electric biking are also great because they exert a large amount of energy, and they can also be relaxing and fun. You can also use a Peloton or another type of indoor bike to use at home instead of going outside for a bike ride. There are a lot of low-impact classes that are easier on the body but will still cause you to break a sweat. The easiest way to build body strength is to do something that you enjoy doing because you will be more motivated to keep going when it feels hard.

Yoga and mat Pilates are also considered strength exercises. They will increase your flexibility and balance while helping you develop calming techniques to improve your mental health. The loss of muscle mass sometimes happens during menopause, which causes balance and mobility to decline. All types of yoga, including hot yoga and traditional yoga, along with Pilates, are very good for your core. Core strength is extremely important because it helps with posture. As we age, we gradually begin to lean forward when we stand or walk because the muscles in our back and core get weak over time. It is not something that happens overnight nor is it something we realize we are doing, but we are not always standing or sitting up as straight as we can. Doing these types of exercises helps strengthen our core and back muscles to support our posture and reduce the risk of falling and a resultant fracture. You have probably heard stories of those who slipped and never recovered. Prepare your body now to reduce your risk.

One of the most important activities to remember to do is to stretch. Stretching should be done before and after every exercise and can even be done on days you don't workout. Your entire body can reap the benefits of stretching. Stretching improves flexibility and increases blood flow to your muscles. It also prevents injury and muscle soreness. Stretching before your workout will increase your performance. It may be tempting to skip the stretch, but even if it is just for five minutes, don't skip it.

Women who consider themselves absolutely fabulous tend to like the way they look. They do not look or feel the way they did in their thirties, but they are happy with where they are now. If they are not, they actively do whatever they feel like they need to do to get there. All of these different types of exercise are good for the body physically *and* mentally. If you do not take anything else from this chapter, remember that you need to move your body. Whatever that looks like for you is up to you, but there is no version of a healthy lifestyle that does not include some sort of exercise. Increasing your individual fitness and well-being might be simply tweaking your regular routine. As you are running those errands, park your car a little further from the door than you normally would. This increases your step count, and it is a small addition to something you are already doing. Just remember to always listen to your body. It is not about being fragile but mindful. If you are unsure about something, talk with your medical healthcare provider first.

TEN

LOVE WHAT YOU EAT

Exercising is not the only requirement for maintaining your physical health. How you treat the outside of your body is just as important as what you put inside of your body. I cannot stress enough how important it is to eat healthier meals. You do not need a dietician or a personal trainer to make better food choices. As we have already discussed, aging naturally brings about a loss of lean body mass, leading to a slower metabolism and making weight loss and maintenance a bit more challenging. Midlife stress makes the issue worse, contributing to the dreaded "muffin top." Being absolutely fabulous means prioritizing mindful eating habits. Start by avoiding eating while driving and instead plan to enjoy all meals while seated and focused. It is easier to overeat if you are not focused on what you are eating. Before each meal, drink 12 ounces of water to distinguish between thirst and genuine hunger. Do not eat if you are not actually hungry. It is not a bad idea to keep your dietary choices private. Some close contacts may inadvertently discourage you. If someone makes a comment on your small lunch, deflect attention by mentioning you had a hearty breakfast.

Address stress or nervous eating habits by engaging in activities like dance classes, cardio workouts, yoga, or Pilates to alleviate anxiety. If you need to soothe your emotions by having something in your mouth, opt for peppermint candy, celery, or affectionate gestures like kissing loved ones. Before attending receptions or events, decide what you will eat beforehand. Choose appetizers like sashimi, chicken, beef skewers, or vegetables without heavy breading or fat content. At a reception, do not rush to the buffet table. When was the last time you went to an event where the host ran out of food? If you can help it, delay eating for 30 minutes while sipping zero-calorie beverages and meeting interesting people.

There is no reason for you to deny yourself the good stuff, so save your calories for indulgent treats like chocolate or whatever your favorite dessert is. You can manage your cravings by allowing yourself a small bite of desired foods and discarding the rest to prevent overindulgence and subsequent guilt. If you happen to overindulge, just love yourself and work out a little more. Whether this way of eating is new or not to you, celebrate each meal's healthy choices to anchor in what you are doing for yourself, and never feel obligated to finish your plate if you are not hungry. Throw it out or take it home. The more you make better eating choices, the better you'll become at knowing just how much food you need to put on your plate. Focus on eating more natural, unprocessed foods. You cannot outwork a bad diet.

If you are trying to control your weight, choose olive oil over butter and limit salt. Eat more healthy fats, lean proteins, veggies, complex carbs, and fruits. Embrace a low-carb lifestyle and weigh yourself weekly for accountability without obsession. This is not about strict rules but more about nurturing a balanced and mindful approach to eating for long-term health and happiness. If you are worried about the number on the scale, do not! Weigh in once a week only. No more, no less. Regardless of what the number says, check in with how you feel. If you feel good, keep going. If not—make some changes. It is true that you only live once, but you also only have one body, so take care of it.

Food plays a crucial part in what's going on with your body. It also plays a huge role in your libido. Even if your hormones are balanced and you find your desire to have sex hasn't returned to where you want it, look at what you have been eating. According to Tiffany Yelverton, Intimacy and Sexual Wellness Advisor, many foods are natural aphrodisiacs that help increase sexual desire and conjure feelings of comfort and safety. Foods like spinach, peanuts, figs, broccoli, and oysters are rich in zinc and regulate prolactin. Avocado and chickpeas are high in Vitamin B6, a libido enhancer. Vitamin C aids in blood circulation and improves testosterone levels— so eat more oranges, yellow bell peppers, and broccoli.

In all of this, whether you are looking to increase your sex life or just how you feel by eating better, do not forget your water. Water intake varies per person, but a good rule of thumb has always been to drink eight cups a day. Hydration plays a key role in your entire lifestyle. If you are dehydrated, your body just won't function the best. Eating better and working out should be long-term lifestyle changes. Everything works together. Balanced hormones, regular exercise, healthy food choices, and managing daily stress reduction boosts metabolism and fosters long-term health benefits.

CHAPTER

ELEVEN

PUT YOURSELF FIRST

One of the best ways to take care of yourself is to put yourself first and do the things you always wanted to do— whether you are married with kids or not. Many women have a list of things they want to try and never get the opportunity to. Sometimes, they didn't because the timing did not work out for them or because they prioritized things like raising their children or other more important obligations. As long as you have breath in your body, it is not too late to start something new. I have a patient who was 68 years old and married for almost 40 years. When her partner died, she was devastated. She was always talking about how sad she was. One day, she picked up bodybuilding because it had always been a dream of hers. Now she is very fit and rocking bikinis every chance she gets. She competes in bodybuilding exhibitions and contests and travels to speak. Of course, bodybuilding is great for her body, but picking it up did wonders for her mind. I am sure she misses her partner, but she's also found a new purpose in the later years of her life. Even if you have to sit down one day and write down all the things you wish you did and still want to do, do it. That will give you a great starting point to start achieving goals that you may have thought were too late for you to achieve.

Putting yourself first and prioritizing the love you have for yourself is a journey, not a destination. It is about taking small steps every day to nurture your mind, body, and spirit. Women need to feel cherished, desired, and adored, and many times, we look to other people for that fulfillment. However, there are plenty of things we can do for ourselves that bring those emotions. It is important to satisfy our fulfillment needs. Whether it is practicing gratitude, setting boundaries, or indulging in some much-needed self-care, prioritize yourself and your well-being. It is easy for a woman to get wrapped up in her marriage or her children's lives. The start of perimenopause sometimes happens at the same time children are getting older and leaving the nest. So, after a woman has had time to balance her hormones and fully embrace the other side of womanhood, she often finds herself with more time and a sense of freedom. Women in their forties and beyond are embracing the beauty of individuality and empowerment and living life on their own terms! Most of my clients are a dynamic group of women, many happily single or with partners with whom they share a peaceful coexistence. For the most part, they are happy. Their children are grown, and they are no longer in the hustle and bustle of school days, leaving them with the freedom to explore personal passions and contribute meaningfully to the world. They already know what it takes to have a happy marriage or relationship. Their priority is being their fabulous and most fulfilled self. Their desire is to find a balance that brings immense joy.

Once you become a woman of a certain age, life is no longer about conforming to societal expectations or focusing solely on relationships. It is about feeling amazing and performing at your best. The emphasis is on mental clarity, quality sleep, positive mood, and a healthy attitude. These women have discovered that the key to radiance is prioritizing self-love and personal growth rather than conforming to outdated norms.

There are so many things you can do that are not just reserved for the younger version of you. You can go to happy hour and grab drinks, attend paint and sips, where you and your friends paint similar pictures, or take cooking classes together. A girls' trip is very good for the soul. In fact, just hanging out with your friends is a great way to unwind. A lot of women are married to older men, and even if they are not, as men age, they do not always have the same energy that their wives do, and sometimes they even prefer to stay at home, but that does not mean you have to.

If your friends are not available, get comfortable with stepping out by yourself as a way to relax. Look up what is going on in your community or a city near you. Festivals are held all throughout the year. Technology and social media bring the world to your fingertips. A quick scroll through your phone will show you lots of things that you can do in your backyard or the backyard of another country you may have always wanted to visit.

If you are not an outdoorsy person, go to the spa or go on a wine tour. When winter comes, don't be afraid to savor the snow. You can get a cabin with a fireplace and enjoy a cozy environment while you nestle in a chair with a hot drink and watch the snow fall. Whether you are hanging out with others or by yourself, look into taking a vacation quarterly. It can be a quick weekend trip or a two-week break. The adventure can interrupt your routine and bring excitement to your life. Your mental health depends on the time you take to reset. Stress can manifest itself in so many different health issues.

You are your most fabulous self when taking care of your body, and you consistently prioritize your health. Many of my clients strive to be the best versions of themselves as they move through the world, whether through impactful careers, community involvement, or personal pursuits. When you are at your best, your world functions at its best.

SECTION 3
FROM THE EXPERTS

REDISCOVERING INTIMACY AND PLEASURE DURING MENOPAUSE

– TIFFANY YELVERTON

A h, the delicate dance of sex and menopause—it is a topic that is often met with hushed tones and hidden embarrassment. But let us face it, it is a conversation that needs to be brought into the light. While this phase can be accompanied by challenges, it is essential to remember that it also presents an opportunity for growth, empowerment, and the reawakening of one's sensuality.

Picture this: you are a woman who has ventured through the perplexing maze of perimenopause and emerged on the other side. While the days of feeling uncomfortable vaginal dryness may be receding, you find yourself in unfamiliar territory. Waning trust in your body's ability to embrace pleasure may be leaving you cautious, timid, and perhaps even hesitant to step into the realm of intimacy and sexual connection.

It would be remiss not to mention the significant role that hormones play in the realm of sexual health. When hormonal imbalances occur, they can significantly impact sex drive and arousal. Balancing testosterone levels can rejuvenate women's sexual vitality, reigniting a passion once thought lost. Upon experiencing hormone balancing, some women describe a newfound sensation akin to regaining a long-lost sense of touch. This restoration of sensory perception is a testament to the intimate connection between hormones and sexual well-being. Rekindling desire can be a gradual process. It is not just a switch that you can turn on once you start feeling things again. It is more like a dimming switch being dialed up. It takes time to nurture and develop those sensations. A lot of women do not realize our genital areas have nerve endings, and when we stop using those nerve endings, they dull out and shut down, just like when you have a cast on your arm, and you do not use it for a while. The tips of your fingers don't feel the same way. So, you must recondition those muscles and nerve endings with exercises like Kegels and massage so that they come back to life.

In addition to the hormones, there are also the mental and emotional pieces. Because of our experiences, some may have built up mental blocks when it comes to sex. I call it the mind, body, and vulva connection. You may hear it called the bio-social-psycho model in other realms. However, my methodology includes more. The emotional, mental, physical, and biological need to be in sync. All of those pieces work together to bring about great pleasure. It is not usually one thing or another. It is not in your mind, and it is not just your hormones causing you to not feel desired or to desire sex. It is more than that. It is the full connection.

The most common concern that women approaching or experiencing menopause seek guidance for is pain during sex. Often, women are told to just drink a glass of wine to relax if the sex is painful. They are told the pain is all in their head. No, it is not. It can be physical. Women can have vaginal atrophy, now referred to as Genitourinary Syndrome of Menopause (GSM), that causes micro tears with penetration, and that is painful. It can also be built-up emotional resentments that are physically causing the vaginal canal to not be susceptible to penetration. That is why it is important to look at the full picture when helping a woman return to experiencing pleasure. Or perhaps experiencing true pleasure for the first time.

The first step towards rejuvenating your intimate life is rebuilding trust with your body. Understanding that your body has changed and learning to appreciate its newness can create a foundation for renewed confidence. Before plunging into the depths of intimacy, take time to reconnect with your body. Begin not with genital touch but with the exploration of your body's landscape. Rediscover forgotten corners, sensitive spots, and areas that ignite a spark of pleasure. Take time to revel in the appreciation of your body in its present form.

The journey to sexual empowerment is not a sprint. It is a tender, patient dance with yourself. By fostering a connection with your body, you lay the foundation for the journey ahead.

Society has ingrained the notion that women's sexual desires wane as they age or that women shouldn't want sex. If we do, then we are a dirty girl. Or we'll ruin our reputation if we have multiple partners. We've been taught that society does not value women who are in tune with their sexuality. However, the work I do every day with my clients challenge that narrative. With my help, women peel back the layers of conditioning and uncover the undeniable truth: women's desires are as potent and multifaceted as men's.

Menopause is an opening act. The layers of societal expectations begin to crumble and reveal an unapologetic celebration of personal agency. Sex gets better with age. It's exciting to see clients in their seventies and eighties flourishing. Sometimes, these women have experienced the death of a partner or have been in a sexless marriage for a long time. And it is not always about intimacy with a partner. It can just be about reconnecting with yourself.

As you step into sexual empowerment after perimenopause, it is an invitation to rekindle the flames that once burned so brightly. Remember, sex can be a fun, healthy, and an exhilarating aspect of life, irrespective of age. Remember the early days of your relationship or when you first met and carry that spirit of discovery into your current experiences. Let go of inhibitions and allow yourself to explore new ways of connecting and expressing affection. Focus on enhancing emotional connection and trust through touch, massages, and exploring one another's bodies.

Do not hesitate, in fact—embrace introducing high-quality lubricants that can enhance pleasure and comfort, ensuring a positive experience for both you and your partner. Just like there are different tools you can use in your kitchen to cook a meal, there are different tools you can use to enhance your sex life, and it can be as good—if not better than before! Sex is not confined to traditional penetrative intercourse. Sex does not have to look the way it looked in your twenties. There is a myriad of ways to experience connection and pleasure. Explore the diverse toolkit of self-discovery using toys, touch, and other forms of stimulation.

Whether you are in a partnership, looking for one, or are content, communication is your greatest ally. Address insecurities openly and find ways to express love, admiration, and appreciation for your partner that transcend physical appearance. If your partner is grappling with insecurities, compliments, praise, and acknowledging their strengths can help bolster their confidence. You are a queen who knows how to make your partner feel like they are ruling the world. Focusing on their love language, be it verbal accolades, engaging in physical touch, spending quality time together, giving gifts, or performing appreciated tasks, can create a positive atmosphere of understanding and trust. Open communication is the cornerstone of any healthy sexual relationship. Contrary to movie depictions, great sex requires dialogue about preferences, boundaries, and desires. Creating a safe space to express needs can transform mediocre experiences into deeply satisfying ones.

I do the work that I do because it is extremely important that everyone has a safe space and the appropriate tools to create the sex life that they truly desire. Once you have had great sex, you always remember it—and desire it. Just like we seek experts to guide us in nutrition, exercise, or menopause, embracing sexual wellness may involve seeking guidance as well. Embracing the journey of self-discovery and prioritizing one's needs contributes to overall well-being and empowerment. Expert advice helps women navigate complex changes, encouraging them to view themselves with love and appreciation.

Yes, there are many things to do and explore on your own. Or you can engage an expert who has been studying intimacy their entire life and has worked with thousands of people to bring back vibrancy. Whether you are looking to start dating in your seventies or you have been married for 50 years, every day can be new and exciting. Of course, you can do all the research and experimentation on your own or simply hire someone to guide you through in a shorter amount of time so that you can obtain results right away.

Sexual empowerment after perimenopause is not confined to the bedroom—it is a radiant force that illuminates every aspect of your life. It is the life force energy that infuses your days with vibrancy, not confined to the parameters of partnered intimacy. The essence of feeling desired, confident, and alive spreads its wings to encompass all that you do. Women often do not realize that when there isn't sexual arousal and those electric feelings in your body, it dulls your entire life, not just your sex life.

Sexual power is not merely about having a partner or engaging in intercourse. It is about nurturing your inner fire and embracing your sensuality. It is the affirmation that your desires matter, regardless of societal expectations or age-related stereotypes. This journey is an evolution—a departure from self-doubt to self-assuredness.

Tiffany Yelverton is the founder and Chief Sexinista of Entice Me Soirees, Inc., and the creator of Sexy Survivors, a digital platform to support female cancer survivors post-treatment. Tiffany is a master at disarming sexual shame and normalizing conversations around sex and pleasure. Tiffany inspires women to love their bodies through self-pleasure and step into their sexual power so that they experience fulfillment in and out of the bedroom. As a quality-of-life sexuality advisor, she facilitates courses, workshops, luxury retreats, and coaching experiences. Entice Me offers a carefully curated line of body-safe, non-toxic sexual pleasure items to enhance life through their network of Sexinistas and online.

Follow Tiffany on Instagram: @enticemesoirees
Visit her website: www.enticeme.com

SEX HORMONE THERAPY

– GAYANE BESNELIAN PHARMD

When we talk about sex, estrogen, progesterone and testosterone are the hormones to pay attention to. Progesterone is the oldest known sex hormone, and it is present in every human regardless of age. It also has receptors in almost all the cells in the body so when there is a decrease in it, a lot of damage can be caused. During menopause, when a woman wants to improve her sex drive, she must look at hormone replacement therapy of all three hormones especially testosterone because it improves the libido. Without it, there is a decrease in the sex drive and a decrease in sexual sensation. Low levels of estrogen can lead to painful intercourse. Low levels of progesterone can lead to lack of sleep, anxiety, and irritability.

As you probably know, women also produce testosterone, just not as much as men. Regardless, it plays a major role in the sex for women as well. In men, the decrease in testosterone can cause an array of unwanted physiological changes. In women it can cause decreased stamina and a loss of sexual interest. Testosterone is also responsible for an increased sense of emotional well-being and since many women are led by their emotions—if they don't feel like themselves then sex is likely the last thing they are thinking about.

As a compounding specialist, I work in a compounding pharmacy where I mix medications specific to a patient's profile. Progesterone cannot be given in pellets so when a patient needs it, a topical cream is offered that can be applied to the inner thigh or the inner arm daily. If the topical solution is inconvenient then there is the option of oral sustained release capsules or vaginal suppositories. The hormones we produce are also yam-based and considered bio-identical because they are as closely related to natural hormones as humanly possible and received very well. If a patient is having trouble with it or not getting the desired results, it is usually a dosing issue and not that their body rejected it. Because testosterone is offered as a pellet, some patients will get a pellet and then a cream or capsule for progesterone. Some patients will try different methods until they find the one that is most convenient for them and also provides the best results.

None of these hormone replacements are available commercially, they must be made at a compounding pharmacy. The key to having successful outcomes is making sure that the patient, the physician, and the pharmacist is involved in the process. Although a patient can come directly to a pharmaceutical office, like mine, to get hormone replacement in the form of topical creams, oral capsules, or vaginal suppositories, they would still need to get lab work done and get a prescription according to their lab results. If they do not have a doctor, then I would refer them to one. A patient can do a saliva test from the comfort of their home and mail it in and then we're able to see what they need in addition to them telling us how they are feeling. I will give them their results and also pass the information along to their physician so that the three of us can discuss the best route to take for hormone replacement therapy. We use this information in addition to the lab work and their doctor prescribes the medication and we fill it. The point of working with a compounding pharmacist, such as myself, and doctors like Dr. Gail Jackson is making sure the dosing is as unique as you are.

Regardless of if a patient elects to do pellets and other solutions, I will always recommend that they see a doctor so that they can discuss all of their options and their well-being in general—not just as it relates to sex. Sex hormone therapy alone isn't always the be all fix-all. To get the most results, you must also change your lifestyle. If you're a smoker, try to stop. It impacts so much more than just your sex drive. Exercising and decreasing your caloric and alcohol intake work together with hormone replacement therapy so that you are functioning as your best self.

Dr. Gayane Besnelian, PharmD is the owner, Chief Executive Officer and Compounding Specialist at Arcade Lane Compounding Pharmacy in Pasadena, California.

Visit her website: www.alcompoundingrx.com
Send her an email to gayane@alcompoundingrx.com
Call her office: (626) 577-7979
Or visit her at Arcade Lane Compounding Pharmacy in Pasadena

ENHANCE YOUR RADIANCE WITH YOUR SMILE

– TONI HENDERSON DDS

A s we age, so will our teeth, and nothing says, "I am old," like yellowed, chipped teeth. There are several ways you can maintain a youthful, more attractive smile. The first and easiest is prevention. Brushing and flossing daily, along with routine dental visits, is a must. Dental checkups and cleanings can detect tooth decay and prevent gum disease. Both ailments, if left untreated, can lead to tooth loss. Missing teeth will cause bone loss and the sinking in of the lower 1/3 of your face, an image we often see on Grandma when she takes her teeth out. Tooth and bone loss will allow tooth movement, creating unattractive, misaligned teeth and harder-to-clean areas and staining. Gum disease can also cause gums to recede, exposing the roots of your teeth and giving you that "long in the tooth" look.

As teeth age, the dentin in our teeth becomes larger, and the enamel that covers it becomes thinner. Dentin gives the tooth its yellow color. Then there is also the staining of enamel over time from the foods and drinks that we consume, such as tomato paste, red wine, and coffee.

Professional teeth whitening, provided by your dentist, can whiten your teeth and bring them back to that brighter, youthful shade.

The wearing of teeth is considered normal as we age. That wear can be slow and even and cause your teeth to become shorter, or it can be extreme and cause chips, cracks, and even movement of your teeth. A good way to prevent excessive wear, which usually occurs at night with clenching and grinding, would be to sleep with a night guard made by your dentist. This appliance will not only prevent your teeth from moving; it will keep your top and bottom teeth apart from each other and, therefore, eliminate possible grinding.

Let us say you have already experienced that darkening and chipping of your teeth, and maybe there has been some tooth movement. If you are a candidate, porcelain tooth veneers could be the answer for you. Picture it as giving your teeth a new face. A perfectly shaped veneer covering your otherwise healthy teeth can give you whiter, perfectly aligned teeth, creating a younger, brighter smile. Veneers are fabricated in a dental lab and will consist of at least two dental visits, making them an expensive option. If veneers are not in your budget, another option could be cosmetic bonding, also known as the poor man's veneer.

Tooth bonding is a procedure in which the dentist will apply a tooth-colored material over the front and edge of your tooth to reshape it and lighten the color. This procedure can be done in one visit and does not require local anesthesia.

So, if you want to keep or create a younger smile, I recommend the following: See your dentist on a regular basis and accept the recommended treatment. Ask your dentist if veneering your teeth with porcelain veneers or in-office tooth bonding is right for you. Add custom-made whitening trays and a night guard to your armamentarium, and do not forget to brush and floss daily.

Dr Toni L Henderson is a practicing General and Cosmetic Dentist in Beverly Hills California, providing dental needs there since 1998.

Visit her website: www.tonihdds.com
Send her an email to tonihdds@aol.com
Call her office: (310) 246-1068
Find her on Facebook: Dr Toni L Henderson DDS
Follow her on Instagram @drtonilhendersondds

LOOKING YOUR
BEST AT ANY AGE
–BLANKA ORLOFF MD

We all want to look our best at any age. Today, modern science offers us preventative and restorative products that help us be our best selves at any age. Taking excellent care of your skin and preventatively avoiding aging stressors will keep the skin looking supple and youthful for a long time.

Sun damage creates free radicals that cause uneven skin color, early onset of wrinkles, and drying of the skin. It is vital to use sunscreen and shield your skin from the sun to keep the skin clear. If you are a smoker, stop. Smoking reduces the blood flow to your skin and can age your skin prematurely. Also, having a skincare routine that hydrates and gently exfoliates your skin can preserve youthful skin for many years. We are all different, and our skin needs differ, too. We all benefit from using products that maintain hydration and exfoliation of our skin.

Other skin care products depend on our own individual type of skin and its needs. The skin care regimen can be as simple as a moisturizer with retinol and sunscreen or significantly more complex. It all depends on how much time one is able and willing to dedicate to one's own skincare. Of course, having regular facials with a qualified esthetician will further deter the aging process and maintain the best skin quality. Modern science allows us to treat many aging conditions of the skin and face, and there are a variety of treatments to address these factors.

Skin tone can often change with time, and uneven skin tone makes us look older. The skin can develop darker spots that can occur from sun exposure, varying hormone levels, physical trauma such as acne or waxing, and other causes. There are a variety of lasers, peels, and depigmenting treatments for each kind of skin type. These processes can be quick, such as a Perfect or TCA peel, or can take longer but have no social downtime like IPL or photo facial treatments. One can develop redness that can be localized to part of the face, like the cheeks, or can be throughout the face. Reducing the redness with a V-beam leads to a more uniform and, therefore, more youthful skin tone.

Worsening skin texture is another aging sign of the face. Acne scars can be treated with microneedling or, in more severe cases, fractional CO_2 lasers. Fine lines around the eyes and lips can be addressed with neuromodulators such as Botox or Dysport. These lines develop from making certain expressions, such as smiling, focusing, and drinking through a straw. By carefully relaxing these muscles, we can soften these lines while maintaining natural movement and softening these wrinkles.

Certain changes occur in the face over time. Our facial skeletons will get thinner and smaller. The eye sockets get larger, and that creates deeper circles under our eyes. We lose the fat in our cheeks, our smile lines become deeper, and we look more tired. Our upper lip slowly rolls "in," and then it thins or disappears.

Today, these changes can be slowed down or even reversed with modern fillers. We can use natural hyaluronic acid fillers such as Juvéderm and Restylane for immediate results, or we can use bio stimulators like Sculptra to create more of one's own collagen and elastin. This process takes longer, but for the client who wants natural results that last longer, this is a great product. Great advances have been made in the field of regenerative medicine, and now one can use one's own blood products, such as PRF or PRP, to restore facial volume and improve the quality of the skin.

We all experience the aging process in different ways, so it is important to develop a relationship with a medical professional who can create a plan specifically for you. A good plan is one that will meet your expectations, is right for your skin type and needs, and fits your lifestyle. The possibilities are endless, but a well-coordinated care plan can keep you looking great for many years.

Dr. Blanka Orloff is passionate about aesthetic excellence and skincare. She has utilized her medical training and background to create and successfully oversee two medical practices, a surgery center (Burbank Plastic Surgery Center) and a medical spa (Skin Matrx Integrated Beauty Solutions).

Visit her website: www.skinmatrx.com
Send her an email to drblanka@me.com

PERFECTLY POLISHED THE STYLE BLUEPRINT FOR HIGH-ACHIEVING WOMEN

– DEANNA DUPREE

"I feel frumpy and matronly."

"I do not want to look like a typical grandmother."

"It is important that my image commands respect."

"I want to feel and look powerful, not too sexy, but in control... and feminine."

"I have never been this size before."

"I do not get the same respect as my colleagues."

"I feel overlooked."

I hear these vociferous whispers from women in leadership so often it hurts. One thing I have come to realize is that there is not enough femininity in leadership. Why? Who said we must look like men in order to do business with them? Remember this, my sweet, YOU are the exception... because you are exceptional! Once you have applied the tips from this yummy chapter of possibility, your peers will find themselves taking a page from your stylebook.

It is totally appropriate to look feminine, sexy, stylish, and professional while feeling sexy and playful. In my opinion, the world needs to see more of it, especially that junior admin who aspires to run her own department or agency. She needs to see you saunter in the office rockin' pearls, a pencil skirt, stunning statement pumps, and a crisp white oxford blouse...with the collar popped, of course (wink!), and a fabulous hobo dangling from your wrist. Do not forget the bold red lip to finish the look. As an Executive Image Consultant and Confidence Coach, I have helped countless high-achieving women elevate their image to non-verbally convey power, brilliance, femininity, self-respect, and sensuality. Yes, sensuality *does* indeed belong in the workplace...especially amongst C-Level women executives.

Many of you are screaming at this page, confused or darn-right in total disagreement with the above statement. Allow me to explain. Sensuality and work are two words that we do not often read in one sentence. Yet connecting our success story and sensuality can be the key to developing confidence to pursue what we want at work— and in life, for that matter. At the same time, this concept goes against what women are taught. Hence, we wonder why we struggle through our work, being exhausted and stressed. As a result of not listening to our heart's desires or prioritizing our pleasures, we are finding more women in leadership overworked, under-dressed, devalued, and overlooked. The primary reason is we have not tapped into our Feminine Power—what we *truly* want and desire. Because *that* power, Beloved, is our source.

The pleasure and joy of a woman are some of the greatest powers that God has given us. It has an exciting effect on herself, her image, her life, and therefore on her work, business, and success. I truly believe if we, the Divine Leaders of the World, begin to dress our Divine Feminine while communicating our desires—we will indeed position ourselves for prosperity and pleasure. As a result, we will invite playfulness and blissful joy into our workplace... and *that* joy **will** spread to every area of our lives.

"Beauty is to recognize how full of Love you are. Sensuality is to let some of that Love shine through your body."
— Nityananda Das, Divine Union

So, how does one incorporate an image of sensuality, power, and respect? You are in the right place, Goddess. It is the Art of Power Play. It is my pleasure to introduce my blueprint for style, sensuality, and business. Here are a few yummy tips to ignite the greatest power that you possess in your work and in your life: Your sensuality!

1. Start each day with a dose of pleasure.

Do something in the morning that connects you with your senses in a pleasurable way, whether anointing yourself with your finest body oils or lotion, sensual dance in the mirror, wearing provocative undergarments, eating dessert for breakfast, wearing lace or silk...or simply doing a short yoga practice (while nude...or wearing your provocative undergarments). Simply stated...anything that makes you feel yummy! Make this part of your ritual or practice to activate your feminine magic, wisdom, and power.

2. Wear something that makes you feel like a Goddess.

After you have activated your dose of pleasure in the morning, use that yumminess to choose ensembles that will radiate and amplify your Power. Now, take a peek in your closet. Notice your favorite blouse, dress, or that item that feels delicious on your skin. Wear that! Wearing something that feels good on your skin, whether it is a pair of pants, a skirt, or a dress, ensures that you can activate your *Goddess Vibes* throughout the day.

3. Have your way with the world!

Put a few reminders in your phone that pop up randomly throughout the day with yummy tasks like "Give someone a compliment, a present, or send a nice message to a friend or colleague." This is my favorite way to flirt!! You'll find the world around you transforming right before your eyes.

4. Communicate your desires by saying, "Yes!"

Although some women are reluctant to ask for a higher price for their services or make the decision for "me time," expressing and communicating your needs and desires are *the most* important things you can do to stay close to your Divine Feminine self and to stay connected with your innate powers. Therefore, train your brain to share its truth by sharing your needs, wants, and desires *every single day*. No matter how small or large.

5. Never blend in.

I am a huge advocate for "Women Against Masculine Pantsuits." No, that is not a real organization, but it certainly should be. You'd find me on the board of directors, for goodness' sake! Instead of "blending in with the guys," consider a marvelous, fitted pant ensemble by Donna Karan or Brandon Maxwell. Very feminine. Very powerful. Remember to go for pops of color, tailor your suits to your frame, and choose exquisite fabrics that transcend time and trends. You'll be sure to slay that next big meeting! Dress your brand, Honey! Increase your demand (wink)!

6. Find your balance.

To achieve a balanced image, you must remember it has a lot to do with the totality of clothes, character, and confidence. Consider my favorite little acronym, which is P.Y.T. (pull yourself together). Remember, power is sexy!

The woman wears the clothes, the clothes do not wear the woman."

My dear, fabulous, sexy Lady Boss...you are MAGIC! You are the Shero we read about in books and magazines. It is high time you dress like it and fully embrace it. This is your time to shine. The world needs more of YOU. Flaunt it, you got it. Dress up. Show up. Stop Hiding.

The fabulous DeAnna DuPree is building brands, confidence, and connections one ensemble at a time. As an in-demand image coach residing in Scottsdale, Arizona, DeAnna empowers emerging executives to dress up, show up, and stop hiding. She also owns a thriving styling studio affectionately named DeAnna's Style Haus, where she creates one-of-a-kind shopping and styling experiences for ambitious women in need of serious playtime.

Follow DeAnna on Instagram: @thefabulousdeannadupree

Join her thriving Facebook Community: facebook.com/groups/impeccablestyle

Visit her website: www.DeAnnaDuPree.com

Send her an email to transform@deannadupree.com

A GUIDE TO PRP THERAPY TO REVITALIZE YOUR HAIR

– JENNIFER SMART-ABBEY MD

As the years go by, many women experience changes in their bodies, and one area that often takes a hit is the health and vitality of their hair. For women over the age of 40, the post-menopausal phase can bring about hormonal shifts that contribute to increased hair shedding and a decrease in hair volume. However, Platelet Rich Plasma (PRP) injections can be a game-changer for your hair by providing a non-invasive way to combat hair loss and boost your confidence.

PRP therapy is an innovative approach that utilizes your body's growth factors to enhance hair growth. PRP injections are known to decrease shedding, stimulate new growth, and increase the diameter of existing hair shafts. Unlike other invasive procedures like hair transplants, PRP therapy is a minimally invasive option with no downtime.

While PRP therapy is a promising solution, it is essential to acknowledge both its advantages and limitations, as it might not work for everyone. It is scientifically proven to be effective for androgenic alopecia (male pattern baldness). However, it can still offer benefits for other forms of hair loss, but results are not guaranteed. Traction alopecia, where there is actual loss of hair follicles, may see less success with PRP. Additionally, individuals with bleeding disorders, autoimmune conditions, or active infections may not be suitable candidates for PRP. Starting PRP therapy earlier in the stages of hair loss tends to yield better results. While it may not be a preventive measure, initiating PRP when you first notice thinning or changes in hair volume offers a higher likelihood of success.

When women first notice hair loss, they often use dietary supplements or vitamins, such as biotin or neutrophil, to support hair growth and retention. PRP therapy, however, adds another layer to this approach. It is not an either-or situation. Women can continue taking their supplements while also receiving PRP injections. While supplements replenish nutrients essential for hair growth, PRP uses the body's plasma to reduce inflammation and stimulate follicles from dormant to active phases. This unique dual-action approach sets PRP apart as a treatment that not only addresses existing hair loss but also encourages new growth as it nourishes the hair follicles.

To assess the extent of hair loss, many women consult dermatologists, who may conduct a biopsy to determine the specific type of alopecia. While a biopsy will provide a definitive diagnosis, it is not necessary for PRP therapy. PRP therapy requires existing hair follicles to work effectively. Even if follicles are dormant, PRP can stimulate them into the active phase, leading to wispy hair growth in specific areas. PRP therapy falls in the middle on the continuum of hair loss solutions, ranging from non-prescription hair serums and prescription foams to more invasive options like hair transplants. Each solution works differently and offers women a range of choices based on their preferences and tolerances. However, a PRP monthly treatment option is less demanding than daily applications of topical solutions but less invasive than surgical interventions.

After the initial sessions, maintenance becomes an individualized choice. Some may find they need less frequent sessions, while others may prefer monthly treatments. PRP therapy allows women to tailor their approach based on their unique results and preferences. The pain associated with PRP therapy is generally well-tolerated. The procedure involves very tiny needles. While some may require numbing cream, the overall discomfort is minimal, and patients become more tolerant of the procedure over time. After the sessions, there is no need to protect your scalp from the sun, but it is advisable to avoid activities like braiding or dyeing your hair for a couple of days. The skin will be tender, but the soreness goes away quickly.

PRP therapy is not a medical necessity for overall health, but its impact on mental well-being should not be underestimated. A woman's confidence is significantly boosted when she feels pleased with her appearance, and enjoying thick, voluminous hair can contribute to a more youthful self-perception. While it might not fully restore previous hair volume, it can significantly improve its thickness and lushness. PRP therapy offers a tangible and empowering choice for women seeking to age gracefully while radiating with confidence and vitality.

Dr. Jennifer Smart-Abbey is a name synonymous with excellence in the field of medical aesthetics. With a profound understanding of the intricacies of the human body and a keen eye for beauty, she has crafted a distinguished career that seamlessly blends science and art. She helps her patients reverse the signs of aging, enhance their features, and embark on journeys of self-renewal.

Conclusion

The journey through perimenopause and menopause is not just a phase of life to endure but rather an opportunity for transformation and empowerment. It is an opportunity to expand into an even better version of ourselves. We recognize and appreciate the paths that have been paved before us, and we also realize the importance of paving a new road for ourselves and the generations that will come after us. This entire book is a love letter to invite you to love yourself more. To put your health first and show up as the best version of yourself— the version of you that is *Absolutely Fabulous.*

The symptoms of perimenopause and menopause once dismissed or silently endured, are now openly discussed and addressed. Through the candid accounts shared in this book, we resonate with the experiences of countless women navigating the challenges of hot flashes, mood swings, and fatigue. It is a reminder that these symptoms are not anomalies but shared realities. Seeking relief is not a sign of weakness but a pursuit of well-being. Balancing your hormones, eating healthier, working out, and doing other things that align with the life you want to live is an opportunity to show yourself the greatest love possible.

As pointed out, traditional Western medicine offers many beneficial solutions, yet it also falls short of providing effective relief for many women during this stage of their life. It is okay to be skeptical, but it is even more important to have an open mind about holistic approaches, like bio-identical hormone balancing, when relief is at the top of your mind. Bio-identical hormone balancing can be a beautiful path to vitality.

The importance of choosing a practitioner with specialized knowledge in hormone balancing cannot be overstated, and I would love for you to pay me a visit. However, as much as credentials matter, so do empathy and understanding. Perimenopause and menopause are vulnerable times because they come from a sense of not knowing what's on the other side or if relief is even possible. This book serves as a beacon of hope for women seeking to reclaim their vitality and embrace the best years of their lives, even beyond the age of fifty. It is a reminder that menopause wellness is not just about managing symptoms but about flourishing in every aspect of life. From medical insights to anti-aging remedies, it offers a comprehensive guide to living the most fabulous life that you can!

As the conversation around perimenopause and menopause continues to gain momentum, this book stands as a testament to the resilience and strength of women everywhere. It is a call to action to advocate for your well-being, prioritize self-care, and embrace the journey of transformation with resilience and grace. Regardless of age, by embracing holistic approaches and making informed lifestyle choices, women can thrive and soar. So, let us embark on this journey together, armed with knowledge, courage, and the determination to live our most fabulous lives.

ACKNOWLEDGEMENTS

This book would be incomplete if I did not acknowledge a few important individuals who made the completion of this manuscript possible.

To my patients, thank you for trusting me with your health. You are the reason I am dedicated to this work, and I will continue working tirelessly to ensure you get the care you deserve. Your stories have inspired me to share this information with the world so other women do not have to suffer needlessly.

To my contributing authors, Tiffany Yelverton, Dr. Gayane Besnelian, Dr. Toni Henderson, Dr. Blanka Orloff, DeAnna DuPree, and Dr. Jennifer Smart-Abbey, thank you. Your willingness to contribute your knowledge is much appreciated. Because of you, this book includes everything women need to know to live their most fabulous lives.

To my book coach and editor, Brittney Smith, thank you for helping me make this dream a reality. Without your guidance and patience, the contents of this book may still be sitting in a folder on my computer.

ABOUT GAIL N. JACKSON MD

Dr. Gail Jackson, a southern girl from Richmond, Virginia, completed her medical education at Howard University before embarking on her obstetrics and gynecology residency training in Los Angeles. She is certified by the American Board of Obstetrics and Gynecology and established her obstetrical and gynecological medical practice at the prestigious Cedars-Sinai Hospital. Dr. Jackson is dedicated to anti-aging and wellness, and her practice offers bio-identical hormone balancing for women over forty using subcutaneous bio-identical hormone pellets. Her vaginal rejuvenation procedure, THE LADYLYFT, and her hormone weight loss and balancing plan, FOREVER FABULOUS, demonstrate her holistic approach to empowering women to embrace life's later chapters feeling confident and vibrant.

Website: www.drgailjackson.com

Email: info@drgailjackson.com

Instagram: @drgailjackson

Made in the USA
Middletown, DE
20 February 2025

71531420R10075